I'm Blessed By God, And
I Have Breast Cancer!

I'm Blessed By God, And I Have Breast Cancer!

"A Journal of My Journey"

Violia Wilson

Library of Congress Control Number:		2012900989
ISBN:	Hardcover	978-1-4691-5386-5
	Softcover	978-1-4691-5385-8
	Ebook	978-1-4691-5387-2

This book was printed in the United States of America.

To order additional copies of this book, contact:
Xlibris Corporation
1-888-795-4274
www.Xlibris.com
Orders@Xlibris.com
110894

Contents

Contents

Dedicated In Memory

of my Mother

Oradell Collins

Who passed away before publishing this book.

Introduction

It never crossed my mind that I'd get breast cancer or any kind of cancer for that reason. It really doesn't run in the family. Maybe just one in every generation got cancer. Well, I guess its numbers are growing.

Everybody was telling me, you'll be all right, you don't have cancer, and the tests will be negative. I was hoping they were right, but I knew the vision God gave me.

I'm just an ordinary Christian woman who loves God with all of my heart and soul. I love God's people and for those who know me, I'd do anything for anybody. God has blessed me with so many gifts and talents that sometimes I'm amazed at what He does through these hands of mine. But to whom much is given, much is required. My life's motto is: *"I can do all things through Christ who strengthens me."* Philippians 4:13. And I have. But facing cancer was the one thing that would make me wonder if I really could do all things. I realized while going through, that it is only with God that I can do anything. And so my faith in God makes me hold on.

I've suffered through most of my life with my health, but I yet continue to work for the Lord. When I was a child I dealt with asthma and severe tonsillitis. I got married to a wonderful man (who is also my pastor) and we had two children. And at age 28, I began a long journey of suffering with ovarian cysts. For almost 14 years, cysts would just burst inside of my belly about 3 to 5 times a year. I'd suffered with extreme pain, total fatigue and infections for about three weeks to a month with each episode. This was a rough time in my life and I thought it would never end. Finally, I received a hysterectomy, and Praise God! It ended all my troubles. So I thought.

After my hysterectomy, I started using a hormone replacement patch to help with the hot flashes and night sweats. I always said, I didn't get hot flashes; I just had one continuous flash that wouldn't quit. After a couple weeks of using the patch, I felt wonderful, hot flashes gone and no night sweats at all. I used that patch for about 3 ½ years and then I found a lump in my breast. Immediately, I stopped using the patch "cold turkey." I took off that patch and refused to wear another. Hot flashes became a part of me. I didn't like it, but what was I suppose to do. No one ever told me of the dangers of the hormone patch.

I had heard on the news that women taking the pill form were getting breast cancer, so I asked my gynecologist about the patch being harmful to me and she confirmed, it was the pill that was causing the problems and that I should be all right. I took her word and well, here's my story.

Violia

1

My Hope

Even before I found out I had breast cancer, God gave me this vision in a dream:

"I was standing on my front porch. There was no door to the outside, just an opening, and I could see everything outdoors. All of a sudden, a horrible storm came up. I'd never seen a storm like this before. It was so destructive, so frightening. I tried to walk toward the opening to the house into the living room, but the wind on the porch was so strong I couldn't move. I literally fell into the wind and it held me up. With every bit of strength I had, I pushed my way toward to the living room, leaning at about a 45 degree angle. I stopped and vomited in a rag that I had in my hand, but I kept pushing with all my might. I finally made it pass the threshold of the doorway. I was almost on the ground but not quite, still held up by the wind. I pulled myself up and looked all around the room and

said, "the house is going to fall," No way would it stand in such a storm! As I walked toward my dining room trying to get away from the danger, I looked all around again, and thought, Oh!, the house <u>is</u> still standing."

Then I woke up.

Immediately I asked God, what was that? What did it mean?" And in a still quiet voice I heard God. He said:

> *"You're going to go through a storm.*
> *It may seem like you're not going to make it*
> *But, The House Will Stand!"*

2

Anticipating The News

It's three days before my surgery and I'm writing in this journal. Not knowing what to expect, I can still hear those words ringing in my ear. Hope from God, that even though I go through, I shall stand.

It was about August/September 2004, I noticed a lump in my left breast. Well for me that was normal. I had small lumpy breast anyway. But this lump didn't dissolve or go away like others had in the past. It became more noticeable and began to worry me. I found myself rubbing that area to see if it would just go away. Finally by the end of October, I scheduled a diagnostic mammogram. An appointment was given to me for early November.

When I went in, I had a regular mammogram and a sonogram. After the tests, the Doctor in the office came in and said he didn't see any significant cyst or tumors on the films. So he sent me home with a peace of mind. But, because I said that I felt a lump, the Doctor found it necessary to check my films more closely using a magnifying glass. (Had I not mentioned that I found a lump, he would have just sent me home and closed my file).

The very next morning, the Radiology clinic called me and asked if I would return and retake more pictures. So I went right in. This time I was a little worried.

They gave me a magnified mammogram and it confirmed my worst fear. Calcifications in the breast that could be cancerous. I left the office with an "I'm Sorry" from the doctor with no further instructions at that point. I was numb!

Later that day my Gynecologist called and recommended I see a surgeon who specializes in care of the breast. She gave me his number; I remember a 410-777-77something. Those numbers alone gave me comfort that God was sending me to the Doctor that He wanted for me. WOW!

I found this Doctor to be a very good and positive Doctor. He was very gentle in his care and he seemed to know just what to say, yet gave all the straight answers to all the many questions I had.

He examined by breasts and without me even showing him where the lump was, he found it himself. He then scheduled me for a biopsy.

3

Caring For Others, Too!

It was near Thanksgiving and God had placed in my heart earlier that year, to have a Thanksgiving Dinner at the church. I could have easily backed out because of my pending health, but I thought . . . Lord, I can cook. I'll feed whoever you send this way, You just take care of me.

So, I went on planning and preparing the dinner and we fed a good amount of people. Even a homeless man who was living in the woods, came in and stayed all day. We were able to find a shelter that would help him too. I wonder, had I been so burdened with my own problems and not prepared that dinner, what would've happened to that man.

God Is Awesome!

A week after Thanksgiving, December 1, 2004, I had my biopsy. I went to The Franklin Square Hospital in Baltimore, Maryland at 8:00 am. I was sent to the Radiology Department. They put me on this table that had a hole in it. My breast went into the hole and a compressor, somewhat like a mammogram, pressed very firmly on my breast so it wouldn't move. I was then lifted toward the ceiling where the technicians could work on my breast under the table.

A needle was inserted, "OUCH!" to numb the breast. Then a drill-like instrument went into the tissue. OUCH! A little more local, and more drilling, OUCH! More medicine, more drilling . . . Ouch! More meds.

After a suction sound, they had some tissue, about the size of a spaghetti noodle in a small container.

I had to lie on that table, breast still compressed while they checked to see if they had enough of the calcifications in that sample. After about 5 minutes, I heard these words . . . "No Mrs. Wilson, we're going to have to do it again. They dialed around to another section and OUCH! Numbing, OUCH, drill, all over again.

Once again, still attached to this table, high up in the air, they checked the second sample. Finally, they said they had enough. After about 45 minutes to an hour, Off came the compression, Ahhh! Relief. Thank God.

I wouldn't know for another week that I would have breast cancer!

4

Surgery

Just before the surgery, a nurse had to inject a dye right into the nipple of my breast in order to illuminate my lymph nodes. The doctor would be removing some of them to see if the cancer had spread outside of the breast. She couldn't give me any pain medication or even do it when I was asleep.

Can you even imagine the pain.

Well, I tell you, I was ready to be put to sleep soon after that procedure.

Surgery went well. "No surprises" at least to the naked eye anyway. I slept most of the day. I was alert around 6:00 pm that evening. Almost 10 hours after general anesthesia. I don't remember anything except my left breast was gone and all bandaged up. I was just numb.

I was given morphine in my I.V. prior to awakening and a little more just around the time I did awake. I tried to tolerate some fluids but began to vomit. Then the nurse gave me some crackers and ginger ale. Still a little nauseated, she called my doctor and he prescribes Reglan. Well, I've had that before and I knew that was it for the day. After the medicine was put in the I.V. and about 30 seconds later . . . I woke up and everybody was gone home. It was about 12:30 am when I looked around and right back out I went again.

About 6:00 am I awoke to the sounds of the Technician waking me for vitals. After she finished, I went into the bathroom and tried to wash up. A struggle, but I did it! I was fit to be tied and got back into my bed. Whew!

From Tuesday to Friday, I experienced no real pain, just some soreness. Saturday came with another chapter, Pain!

5

Nothing Like Family

Unless you have a family like I have, you'll never know the real blessing of their existence. My mother, Oradell, who was sick herself and recovering from surgery in November, would have been at my house when I came home from the hospital, but I told her not to worry and to stay home. But I know she had fasted and prayed for me the day of surgery and continued to pray for my healing daily.

My youngest sister, Veronica, took care of me that first week. From nurse duties to cleaning house, she did it all. She would arrive early at 8:00 am every morning and literally stayed all day until about 9:30-10:00 pm.

She fixed my breakfast, cleaned my bed, laid out my underwear and gowns, cleaned my bedroom, while Tia, my daughter, and I took a shower. I needed much help and Tia got right in and washed me, dried me and put lotion on me and helped me to get dressed.

Veronica cleaned my whole house, scrubbed floors, washed my clothes, fixed my lunch and dinner and fed my family; she gave me snacks in between my meals and gave me my medicines. She stripped and emptied my drains several times a day and I'm sure she did things that I don't even know about, but was necessary. All I know, she took wonderful care of me and my family for 7 days. And on the 8th day she had to return back to her own job. But she called me and checked on me around lunch time and brought me dinner every evening. How blessed am I.

My oldest sister Vanessa is definitely a prayer warrior. Whatever I or anyone in the family goes through, we can rest assure that Vanessa is praying for us. All of my sisters and I are very close and they just stuck together with me throughout this sickness. Verneice, my next to the youngest sister stopped in and gave a helping hand as well. Whatever I needed, the sistas made sure I had it.

Thank God for family. I'll tell you more about them later.

But the news I received on that day, stunned everyone.

6

Even More Bad News

I found out that the cancer was found in my lymph nodes. Ratios of 8 out of 10 were cancerous. I was at stage 3, Not good! My doctor wanted me to go to see an Oncologist to seek treatment by Chemotherapy.

Chemotherapy! The one word I didn't want to hear. But now I stood face to face with this demon.

This too shall pass.

As I recline in the arms of my heavenly Father, I know still, "The House Will Stand!"

My first visit to the oncologist was a very long and extremely stressful event. The doctor talked with my husband Doug and I and told us what to expect. It was such an overwhelming amount of information, that when I left the office I actually felt nauseated.

I was absolutely sick to my stomach with grief and I literally shook all over. I looked at Doug and said, *"I can't do this."* I just wanted to give up. He, being as compassionate as any man could be, assured me I can do this. In fact, he said. *"We can do this."* Never did he separate himself from this disease as my problem. It was always our problem. Praise God for this man. His love still helps me day by day.

The oncologist wanted me to have a PET Scan done the very next day. The appointment was made and I went in the next morning. Well, inside of that tunnel, I panicked. I've had CT scans before, what made this different? I just totally lost it. I prayed and asked God to please help me through. I tried to think of just one song to hum. Couldn't think of nothing. I tried praying for my family; the quickest prayer ever. I tried everything I could think of at that moment (which wasn't much) but I kept getting overwhelmed. Finally, I was pulled out of the machine. Thank you, Jesus! I was fit to be tied again. Soaked from sweat and fear, I went home and had to change my clothes. Whew! This journey is only the beginning. *"Oh Lord, please help me through."*

Later that day I had an appointment with an image recovery center in Baltimore, located at the Harry and Jeanette Weinberg Cancer Institute at Franklin Square. I found this center to be most informative for patients with cancer, whether they were still receiving treatments for chemo or after treatment was done. I was able to pick out a wig for when I lost my hair, and buy special skin and personal products especially designed with the chemotherapy patients in mind.

Every time I visited the center I would leave lifted up and feeling a sense of going on. I'd recommend every cancer patient to find one of these centers in their area. It was truly uplifting for me, knowing that there are things I can do to help me as I go through, to look and feel my best. They answered so many of my questions and fitted me for a mastectomy bra, as well as ordered a custom made breast prosthesis.

This place made me smile.

7

Surgery Again

A second surgery was scheduled for me to get a port-a-cath put in. This would keep my veins from collapsing or being used up. The chemo would be done right through this port under the skin in my chest. This was a minor surgical procedure done as an outpatient in the hospital.

This surgery was probably one that most people wouldn't want to experience. "The Nightmare of Surgery." I guess you're wondering, what is the Nightmare of Surgery? Answer: Waking up while the operation is still going on.

Yes, right in the middle of surgery I just woke up. Ouch! The pain of somebody tinkering around in your neck and chest . . . well, you get the picture. These are the times I wish I could just pass out. Unfortunately, I had all the sleep I was going to get for a while. The Doctor finished the surgery and they lifted me off the table and rolled me into recovery, and yes, I was still awake.

I was given morphine, and some kind of muscle relaxer, then another pain medication. I felt so nauseated from being highly medicated, that all I could do was vomit. I was given my instructions and out the door I was sent, very quickly.

When I arrived home, I was just so sick. My husband Doug and sister Vanessa helped me out of my clothes and into my gown. I remember easing down on my pillows and out I went.

The rest of that day I spent vomiting and sleeping. What a day!

My next hurdle, Chemo!

"Father in heaven, as I get closer to receiving Chemotherapy, I ask as one of your children, to be the exception to every rule of man. When men say I'll be sick, make me well, when men say I'll be weak, make me strong. In my life Lord, be glorified today." A-men

8

Anxiety

Another demon to contend with is Anxiety (That feeling of being closed in or trapped). Every now and again this guy creeps up on me and just overwhelms me.

Sometimes I look too far ahead and get overwhelmed. I used a metaphor once in a Children's Ministry class and often shared with others, that we only have a snapshot (today), God has the whole roll of film. If we try to see the whole film it will be overwhelming. So we must just look at the snapshot of the present, and only focus on what's facing us today. Just one day at a time. In time God will unroll the whole film and when we look back, we can see where He's brought us through.

"Thank you Lord, for Today!
However crazy a day it might be,
I know You can take me through.

Yesterday's fears are behind me
never to bother me again.
Tomorrow is yours to guide me, and until
then, I'll face that day when it comes.
But right now, today Oh Lord I pray,
help me to make it through."

Doug is probably the best husband on earth. He is just so caring and wonderful. He is the man that holds up the wedding vows, for better or worst, in sickness and in health, always keeping us as one.

Whenever anxiety would arise, I could call him and he would come and just hold me and talk to me. He would tell me how much he loved me and how thankful to God he was for me. It wasn't long before I began to feel better again. I don't know if I could go through without him and I don't want to find out.

Mom always checked in with me every day. If I told her I felt a little anxious, well, before the day was over the whole family was there making me laugh, bringing food, praying, singing and just being what family is all about. I have the best family too.

"Thank you Lord, for my wonderful family."

One day at a time with God, and family, I can make it.

As I'm writing this journal, I am yet going through. I wait one more day before Chemo begins. But God has me in His loving arms.

9

Chemo, In All It's Glory

Well, The day came and has gone. Today is the third day after Chemo. I can't think of words to describe the last couple of days. On the day of the Chemo, I felt okay, and tolerated the fluids and the many Medicines I was given that day. One of the main chemicals was Adriamycin & Cytoxan (A/C). These are what effects the hair, nails and skin. Later that evening I started feeling a little nauseated as well as during the night. The next day I had to go back to the clinic for fluids and some more medicine. I wasn't feeling my best but not too bad either. The Latter part of day two, I was just sick. Very nauseated and feeling low energy, I kept pushing myself to do whatever I needed to do, but I really couldn't do too much.

By day three, I woke up shaking all over. My glucose level was very low. A little food and orange juice helped to bring that up. I just felt sluggish, slow and out of it. But God is yet carrying me through.

From around the 3rd day after Chemo to about the 8th day, I was just sick and nauseated. I couldn't eat much at all or even talk to anyone. I just groaned and shook my head yes or no. Just so very sick.

After the fifth day I started feeling better each day that followed. I had my blood work on Thursday and it was very good. My red blood cells were up and I didn't have to get a shot.

"Praise the Lord, for He is good and His mercy endureth forever!"

My 2nd Chemo went well. I felt pretty good. By now my finger nails and nails on my feet had turned black from the chemicals. My skin was a grayish tone. I looked dead, but my Doctor said my blood tests was unusually good for someone going through Chemo. I knew that "unusually good" is how God deals with us in a bad situation. Just what I prayed for; the exception to the rules of man. He is carrying me through.

So many prayers yet going up for me, and so many blessings yet pouring upon me.

"Thank you Father!
And thank you for showing me that so many people
really love and care much about me."

10

The Hair Cometh Out

The next morning I noticed a little hair on my pillow. I reached up and gently pulled my hair and long strands just came out. I got up and started to comb it and you just wouldn't believe the clumps of hair. Yes! "The hair cometh out!" I took a little clump of hair and tied a band around it tightly and cut it off for my husband Doug. He just wanted to save it I guess. Anyway, the more I combed or brushed, the more clumps came out, so I decided to just go and have my head shaved. 46 years of having hair and lots of it, sure is going to feel different. But stress is not a part of me today, for I am alive. My hair will grow back someday and like the character "Job," in the Bible, it will be doubled.

My daughter and I went to the Cancer Center and she watched, teary eyed, as the technician shaved all my hair off. At that point it really didn't bother me, somehow I knew my hair was going to come out and I was okay with that.

I brought a nice wig, sort of a honey color. I figured if I'm going to change, I may as well go drastic. But it looked very nice with my complexion, everybody liked it and so did I. So, with less time to do my hair, I now have more time for other things.

When I came home with my perfect little round bald head, my family kept telling me I was beautiful. It made me feel good, because what I saw in the mirror was not so beautiful to me. But it was me, bald, gray with black nails and I was alive.

The following week, I was just nauseated the entire week up to the next Chemo session. Rough, rough, rough, that's all I could say. Each session seemed to be different and more intense than the others.

11

I Feel Like Going On

My lovely daughter Tia, is getting married in August. God has blessed me with many talents and I had planned to do everything for her wedding. I mean literally everything! But sometimes our plans get a little sidetracked.

At first I wondered why this had to happen at this time in my life. I had made many wedding dresses for many young ladies in the past, and here I was facing the fact that I might not be able to make my own daughter's wedding gown. But I realized as I'm going through, that there are no give-up days in this fight. You have to be positive and want to survive, always. I believe that God knows how strong-willed I am about doing anything. He knows that when I start something, I don't stop until I'm finished and it's done right. He knew I would push hard so that I could make Tia's dress, her bridesmaids and flower girls (10 all together) for her wedding, and all the decorations and flowers as well. This was enough to keep me going beyond my finish date of Chemo.

And as I have found out in the past, in my weakness God is most strong. So I anticipate what God will do through these hands of mine. And I give Him all the glory right now for what He will do.

During the first few days of treatment, I'd rest and do very little, but the week after, I would sew or make something. God is Awesome. By the time of my 2nd Chemo I had reached a goal that I set for myself to have at least the bridesmaid dresses cut. And I did!

All 7 were cut and hanging up ready for me to sew as soon as I felt better the next go round. After I finish sewing them, I'll cut out the two flower girl dresses and sew them (2 more down). I probably won't start Tia's gown until June when I finish Chemo. But who knows what God has in store for me. He is Just Awesome.

A song that has been on my heart lately was . . .

"I feel like going on, I feel like going on,
Though trials come, on every hand,
I feel like going on."

And yes, I do feel like going on!

12

Eggs, Eggs and More Eggs

Eating is one of the important things you must do while on Chemo and probably the most difficult thing to do. This is no time to diet! You must eat to keep up your strength and give your body a fighting chance. *"That's a big joke!"* I thought. Eating was far from my mind on those bad Nauseating days. All the foods I used to eat, I couldn't stomach at all. I didn't want anything to eat. All I wanted to do was rest.

The only thing that I could eat and I craved them everyday were eggs. Fried egg sandwiches, scrambled eggs, eggs with cheese, eggs in salad . . . Didn't matter how they were fixed, I had to have one every day.

My husband became quite the gourmet egg preparer. He made an egg sandwich that was out of this world. yummmm. I looked forward to them everyday. It was just about the only food I could tolerate on those Chemo days and the week following.

Come to find out, the Doctor said "The best thing for me to eat now was eggs. Wow! My body knew that.

How awesome are You dear Lord.
You have made us and we are wonderfully made.

13

More Chemo

The third Chemo treatment was the beginning of an interesting week. By Friday, I was just so ill. I had absolutely no strength in my body. I woke up and went to the bathroom to brush my teeth and shower. By the time I came out of the bathroom, all I could barely do is put on another gown and literally fall back into bed. I could not sit up or even move.

One day my husband was attending a Good Friday Service, Tia was at work and Dougie (my 25 year old son) was the only one at home with me. When it comes to me being sick, Dougie has no idea what to do. Dougie is one of those laid back, care free individuals who just happens to live in my home. He's a very caring person and wonderful child. But one thing he always liked to do is call 9-1-1.

I told him I wasn't feeling very well and couldn't get my food or medicine. Well, he called in the troops, "My Family." Veronica was at work, but her husband Bobby (who is a EMT) showed up in a matter of minutes. In emergencies we always call on Bobby whenever he is available. Soon behind him was my mother and sister Vanessa. Even Justin, my favorite great nephew (and only one) came to cheer me up.

Mom fixed the ever-unchanging egg sandwich and some orange juice. I was able to eat and take my medicine, but I stayed in bed all day and all night. By Saturday, I was still a little tired but Tia woke me up with my egg sandwich and meds. After my shower, I laid down for a little while and got up later. Plopping from chair to chair. I could only just rest in Jesus. Whew! this Chemo can wear you down!

Nausea continued through the weekend but by Monday I started to feel better with each passing day. By Wednesday, I didn't have to take any more of the nausea medicine and I actually felt pretty good by the weekend. I ate pretty good and even tried a few new things in my diet. I felt great!

The weather was warm and I wanted to work in my garden. My husband and I brought a few early plants and planted them outdoors and I started my yearly herbs in peat pots indoors. I was doing just fine and then . . . Chemo #4.

Same ole same ole, yucky feeling and days waiting to feel good, but even in my distress, God is yet carrying me through. Sometimes I want to just give up, but I can't, I must go through. I'm halfway through the Chemo now. Eight more weeks to finish, I can make it! With God on my side I can make it, one day at a time.

14

Chemo Times Two

The second half of Chemo (the last 8 weeks) is another mixture of medications ending with the main medicine, called Taxol. This medication, or should I say "Chemical," effects the bone in the body.

It, like the Adriamycin & Cytoxan (A/C) which affects the hair skin and nails, goes to another extreme.

I didn't experience the nausea like with the A/C, in fact, my appetite actually got better, but the extreme nausea that I felt while on the A/C, was felt in pain with the Taxol.

"I never felt felt, that felt like that felt, felt, before." (say that fast 3 times)

The pain that racked my entire body was so intense that my body would literally convulse as if I were being shocked by electricity. My muscles would flinch all over. Every part of my body hurt. My teeth hurt, my spine, my thighs, knees, legs and feet. The very bottom of my feet hurt so badly that I could hardly walk.

My hands hurt, my neck and head, just everywhere.

For about 5 days after Chemo I would experience great pain. After about the fifth day, the pain would ease up a little each day. (Praise God!) By the end of the week I would start to feel better, then, it was time for Chemo again. After the second treatment of Taxol, my feet wouldn't get better. Each Chemo thereafter left my feet and hands with neuropathy (numbness and tingling) in them. Even now I suffer with this affliction. I don't know when it will go away, but my prayer is that God will heal me from it.

Four treatments of Taxol, and with each treatment, the pain was more severe than the last treatment.

We can never know how great God is unless He takes us through such great pain. This pain was so great, that for me, it was a miracle to get relief. *"Thank You, Lord!"*

I thank God for my praying husband. When I would flinch in pain, he would anoint me with oil and pray for me. Sometimes the pain would just over whelm me so, that I didn't know what to do, and he would just pray. The expression on his face was as if he could feel my pain. Just having him there helped me to bear a lot of my pain. Oh how I thank God for my husband. Even in Pain, God is Just soooo—Good!

With numb hands and feet, I began and finished my daughter's wedding gown. With God doing all the work through these troubled hands of mine, I'm amazed at the results. I knew He would do a better job than me anyway. *"Thank you, Lord, because in my own power I could have done nothing."* But with God, I not only finished her wedding gown, but I had finished all 10 of the gowns, all 10 bouquets, the pew bows, arch and decorations, the flowers, the invitations, the programs, the mini newspapers and everything else I needed to do.

Even with Cancer . . .

"I can do all things through Christ who strengthens me."
God is Awesome!!!

15

Radiation

Approximately 3 weeks after I finished Chemo, I began my radiation treatments. Radiation would kill any abnormal tissue left in the body that chemo may have missed. My treatments were scheduled for 6 ½ weeks, Monday—Fridays. It was like getting an x-ray only the dose was longer and higher. I had 4 different positions of radiation. It took about 10 minutes or so to do (whenever the machine acted right). So, I was in and out usually in about 30 minutes each day.

So, on June 20, 2005, I began another unknown journey. The weather was hot and being radiated for 33 days from June to August (not counting the weekends) was really something to deal with. Kinda like being microwaved on a hot Island.

They laid me down on the table and literally mark little x's and lines on my skin with permanent markers, so that I would be positioned exactly the same each time I went for treatments. Afterwards, they actually gave me real tattoo dots to make those marks permanent. The aim of the equipment had to be just right so the radiation would miss damaging my heart and lungs, so those markers had to be there for my safety.

At first I felt nothing but a little tired. Then after about 1 ½ weeks, I started noticing that my skin from under my arm to the center of my chest becoming pink, very pink. I guess the radiation was working. I was given an ointment to apply during the day after my treatments. It helped to keep my skin moisturized so it wouldn't peel or open up. I even noticed slight burning on my back. The radiation was penetrating all the way through me.

After about 3 weeks, my skin was purple and quite sore. I continued using an ointment that was suggested by a friend, 100% Aloe Vera Gel. She told me to keep it in the refrigerator. This really helped me a lot.

Have you ever burned yourself badly and the burning sensation was still there hours later? That's what my skin felt like, only times 100 and it pained me for days. That cold Aloe really gave me relief. Thanks Diane!! (a wonderful friend who went through cancer and many other sickness' and finally *"won the fight"* and is home with Jesus now!) Notice I said "won." So many people say . . . they lost their fight with cancer, but with Jesus, it's a win, win situation.

The sixth week of Treatment was rough. My skin was extremely sore. I had blisters that popped and oozed. My skin was badly burned and almost black. My chest felt tight like someone had tied a belt around me. As I approach the end days of radiation, I wonder, with my 3rd degree burns if I would even be able to wear a dress at my daughters wedding.

Finally, the end! I'm finished radiation and I'm as sore as can be, my skin is peeling severely, leaving that raw, pink. and overly sensitive skin exposed. (yuck) The Doctor prescribed a cream used for burned patients called Silvadene, which is used for raw inflamed skin. I can't do hardy anything without causing pain in that area. So I just try to sit still with my arm propped up and my head to the side.

Very quickly, I learned that Silvadene is a product that actually has silver in it, which I am allergic to, so on top of the raw inflamed tissue, I broke out in an awful blistering oozing rash. What a mess! I had to use an antibiotic ointment and another petroleum ointment and I kept my skin covered with fresh gauze daily.

But, I'm still alive and God is yet in control of my life. I am blessed and highly favored by the Lord. Some may think, "How are you highly favored of the Lord and having to go through so much."

The very fact that God showed me and told me that I was going to go through a storm and then it happens just as I was told, shows me His favor. God called my name. Wow!

16

Wedding Jitters . . .

As I approached 2 weeks before my daughters wedding, I was still very sore and raw. I prayed for a great Wedding Day and ceremony and that my pain would be gone and that I would be able to enjoy the day's festivities. I worked on a power point for my daughter's wedding to be shown at the reception. Even sitting at the computer was a task with great deal of discomfort.

On the morning of my daughter's wedding it was raining just a little. We arose early so that I could do her hair. A beautiful bride indeed and she didn't even have her dress on yet.

A little while later a rainbow appeared in the southern sky of our sunroom door. I told my daughter that the day would be all right, that the rainbow meant the storm was over. She smiled and said, "Mom, maybe this rainbow was sent for you. Your storm is over."

I thought about it and she was right. My storm was over, Praise God!

> **Whatever your cross, Whatever your pain,**
> **There will always be sunshine, After the rain . . .**
> **Perhaps you may stumble, perhaps even fall,**
> **But God's always ready, To answer your call . . .**
> **He knows every heartache, Sees every tear,**
> **A word from His lips, Can calm every fear . . .**
> **Your sorrows may linger, Throughout the night,**
> **But suddenly vanish, Dawns early light . . .**
> **The Savior is waiting, Somewhere above,**
> **To give you His grace, And send you His love . . .**
> **Whatever your cross, Whatever your pain,**
> **"God always sends rainbows . . .**
> **After the rain . . ."**
> *Author Unknown*

And the wedding was absolutely Awesome!

17

Conclusion

You never know in life, which way your life will go. We can try to make what we think is a better decision, but we will ultimately end up exactly where God wants us to be.

Sometimes we worry too much about doing everything just right; having what we think is *"A Perfect Life."* But, a wake up call is coming to us all. Life isn't about being perfect in the eyesight of others; it's about serving a perfect God and allowing His perfect-ness to work in our imperfect life, making us instruments of His service, sharing the Gospel with everyone that we meet in life.

Life is family, friends and loved ones. No need to fret about things being just right. "I'm Alive, and all is alright."

I may be a little disfigured, but I'm able to hug my husband and children and my beautiful granddaughters). I can still show love to my friends and church family and all who come in my life.

The doctor told me, that while I was receiving Chemo; my liver functions were extremely low, in fact critical. Many patients don't make it through Chemo because the Chemo would cause death and not the cancer itself. He never said anything to me about this until a year after my Chemo, when my numbers were up. He said he didn't want to put any more on me since I was being treated with extremely high doses of Chemotherapy (16 weeks). He just watched me closely hoping I'd make it through. And now, I can look back and know that I was truly in the Hands of God, for it could only have been Him that brought me to where I am today . . . Healed.

As this book is being published, I'm now seven years cancer free and to anyone who may be going through your storm, know that God can do anything. My faith kept me going each day and it still keeps me going today.

I'm healed and I praise God with everything that I am. I know it's Him who keeps me everyday. And I know it will be Him who takes me through this life.

"Thank you Father, for working through the hands of the Doctors, Nurses and everyone that you've put in my life, who helped me. You deserve all glory, honor and praise and I Love You, Lord!"

I had cancer, but . . . "The House Is Still Standing!"

If you must go through, You too, can make it. Trust God! Be sure to get your yearly mammogram and it's a must that you do self exams every month. Remember, I found a lump from a self exam. My mammogram did not show the calcifications until they magnified it. They only magnified it because I had said, "I found a lump." Be Blessed and take care of yourself.

Website Information: If you would like to view the pictures of my daughter's wedding and all of the accomplishments that I was able to do while going through Chemotherapy and Radiation, check out my page on facebook:

http://www.facebook.com/pages/Violia-Wilson/231574673587228?sk=wall

See how God used me during the sickest time of my life, and He can do the same for you. I am truly blessed by God!

www.ingramcontent.com/pod-product-compliance
Lightning Source LLC
Chambersburg PA
CBHW021302280526
45784CB00005B/2479